Dedication:

This book is dedicated to my lovely wife – Tessa McNeal. Without your love and support, I would not be able to be the man that I am. I definitely would not have as much enjoyment in my life without you. I would also like to thank my family both in the Philippines and the United States. Thank you for your support, encouragement, and understanding. Praise God and give God all of the glory. Without him nothing is possible but through him all things are possible. Thank you, God, for allowing me to write this book.

Copyright and Terms

Copyright © 2020 by Rational Solutions, LLC
All rights reserved.
Expanded Print Edition v1.1

ISBN: 9798654310583
Imprint: Independently published

Disclaimer Note

This program contains exercises that, depending on your physical condition, may be hazardous to your health. Consult with your doctor before attempting these exercises. It is also important that you use care in performing the exercises in this book, since improper performance could result in injury.

The user of this book, and the information contained in this book, assumes all risks for performing the exercises described in this book. Use of this book constitutes a covenant not to bring any lawsuit or action for injury caused by performing exercises described in this book.

Table of Contents

Introduction

Congratulations! You are well on your way to building the sleeve busting muscular arms that you have always wanted. My program works, but it comes at a price. I'm not going to lie to you and tell you that it is super easy, because it isn't. I'm also not going to tell you that you can sit on your butt and meditate about the meaning of the universe and automatically build strong, powerful arms. Finally, I'm not going to tell you that you can eat some magic pill composed of nutrients found in mold spores from a mythical rain forest to jack up your arms.

Those would be lies, and that would be crap that doesn't work. My program works but it requires your dedication, and it requires a lot of hard work. You will be sore, and this program will make you tired, but the results will be worth it. In 30 short days or about 8 workouts you can gain serious permanent size to your upper arm mass. It is that simple.

Do the work = Get the results.

My book is inexpensive because I want to share it with you. I know that you will get the results that you want, and that is all I want for you. I want you to be successful.

This program is so effective because it utilizes multiple muscle-building strategies and techniques that function synergistically to optimize and activate the most amount of muscle fiber in every workout.

This program uses muscle-building techniques that have existed for some time, but it is the unique combination of these techniques that make my program so effective.

Many of the exercises in this book, you may be familiar with, but it is the unique timing, rep count, sequence, exercise selection and technique that make my program so effective.

I can't tell you how pleased it used to make me to have people stop and stare at my arms whenever I was shirtless, or I was wearing a muscle shirt. I even had one guy tell his friend that if his arms looked like mine, that he would wear a muscle shirt too. Those were my egotistical younger days however, and I will leave those days to the younger men. I am married now and not interested in having huge guns to attract the girls.

Now I just try to find comfortable clothing that fits me properly. That is a real struggle because of my size. My arms are now about 20 inches around, but the largest they ever were was 21 inches. That was really the largest that I ever wanted or needed. You may be different, and you can continue to use this program to keep packing on permanent size as needed up to your genetic potential.

I want to make it clear that I am not a doctor or exercise physiologist, and I don't play one on TV, but I do believe in this program. After you finish this program, you will be a believer in how effective it is too.

Always check with your doctor before beginning this or any exercise program.

Before we get into exactly why this program works, I want to provide you with some terminology that will be used throughout this book.

Hypertrophy:

An increase in muscle mass or girth of a muscle that is induced by an external stimuli such as resistance training or when doing progressive overload training, which causes the body to respond by pushing healing nutrients into the affected area to initiate healing (growth).

Microfiber tears:

Muscle growth is initiated from extremely small (micro) tearing of the muscle fibers. The body adapts to this "injury" by attempting to heal itself. With proper rest and nutrition, new muscle fibers form between the old ones, which leads to the growth of bigger and denser muscle. My program incorporates the maximum possible amount of muscle fibers, which means that you will tear/breakdown more muscle fiber then you normally would. Which will cause you to grow bigger and stronger once your body heals/adapts.

Muscle-activation:

The process of recruiting specific muscle fibers and the central nervous system in performing an exercise; the muscle must "fire" in order to perform the exercise successfully. The more muscle activation that occurs during an exercise set, the higher the amount of microfiber tears that can occur resulting in maximal muscle hypertrophy.

Exercise selection:

I've selected exercises in this program that compliment and increase the amount of muscle activation by set. For example, when you work the bicep you also work the brachialis. Therefore, I work the bicep heavily, and then we go directly to movements that also stress the bicep but dig deep into the brachialis, and brachioradialis (forearm muscle). Stacking exercise selections like this create a synergistic effect, which overloads each muscle in the chain. Recruiting more muscle fibers to shock the muscle into growth.

Progressive overloading:

In order to increase the strength inside of a muscle and to grow the muscles; the muscles need to be overloaded, which stimulates the natural adaptive processes of the human body, which develops to cope with the new demands placed on it.

Progressive overload stimulates muscle hypertrophy, and it also stimulates the development of stronger and denser bones, ligaments, tendons and cartilage. Progressive overload also causes increased blood flow to the region of the body that is being worked. Finally, progressive overload stimulates the development of more responsive nerve connection between the brain and the muscles involved. That nerve connection means that your body will become more efficient at performing the exercise over time and that means that you will become stronger at that movement.

The Science

This program works. I have used this system on trainee's dozens of times since its development and I have always had great results. In 1998, I had the opportunity to train a member of the United States Army. I will call him David. David was a classic hard gainer, tall and lanky. No matter what he did, he couldn't gain weight or muscle and had abysmally small arms at just 11 inches in circumference. Just to put that into perspective, the average adult male's arm circumference is 13 inches.

David had such a hard time gaining muscular weight that he had been placed in the Army's weight control program to help him increase his weight. David was 5' 10" tall and weighed 135 pounds. The military's program succeeded in only keeping David at his current weight and kept him from losing weight during the intense training sessions the military requires. I placed David on this program and worked out with him every week. He lived with me at the time and followed all of the advice that I gave him. We worked out on a 4-day per week schedule, separating workout days into two categories of lower body and upper body. We utilized mass building compound exercises including deadlifts, shrugs, pull-ups, military presses, squats, and the bench press. He did this arm workout on upper body days and only this workout for his arms.

In only 1 month, David had gained 15 pounds and several inches over his entire body. His upper arm measurement was 13 inches and had clear definition. Let me be clear, he was still very lean, but had added several pounds of muscle to his frame.

David followed my dietary guidelines and woke up at 3:00 am every morning for a protein shake before going back to sleep. He ate a lot, and worked his butt off, but in the end his hard work paid off in fantastic results. David is now able to maintain a healthy weight.

Timing

Resting too long between sets of exercise and performing the repetitions of an exercise too slowly will stifle your muscle growth. My program eliminates rest completely so that the muscle group is extremely fatigued. This causes the body to sense additional stress that it may not feel otherwise. This is also why you have to use less weight on my program than what you may be used to.

Range of motion

My program uses a full range of motion on most exercises to completely exhaust as much of the muscle as possible. This allows you to activate more of the muscle than you might normally in a standard weight-training program.

Training stress

Stress before training is very low, but during training the stress rises to a high level that is based on the amount of exertion or effort you are putting into each set. At the end of a set, the stress starts to decrease again, and if given enough time would return to the starting stress level. My training program alters the exercise sequence to trick the body into continuing the exertion and the muscle activation. This causes more muscle fibers to fire, and the stress to increase. This essentially panics the body into responding with accelerated muscle hypertrophy.

Muscular tension/confusion

Everyone knows that in order to get stronger, you have to lift heavier weights and for the most part that is true. However, you must also effectively target the appropriate weight throughout the strength curve. The strength curve is basically the point, during a movement, when the muscle is capable of producing different levels of strength. My program uses this principle coupled with alternating sequences of high and low repetitions to keep the muscle under maximum stress throughout its movement. Additionally, by varying the tension, workout to workout, the muscle is forced to adapt more rapidly because it increases the muscle confusion.

Let me give you a quick example. A carpenter swings a 16-ounce hammer for long periods throughout the day. At first a new carpenter may experience soreness in his/her arm from that movement and those repetitions. However, his/her body responds to this stress and muscular tension by getting stronger. That is adaptation, and the reason why carpenters don't typically continue to grow and get stronger and stronger. Their body adapts to the stress and stops growing. However, my program does not allow your body to fully adjust so your body must continue to adapt by getting stronger and bigger. That is known as muscle confusion.

The end result

The Massive Biceps and Triceps program that I have developed is structured to maximize the training stress, the muscular tension/confusion, the timing, and the range of motion during each portion (Biceps and Triceps) and will allow you to achieve maximum muscle growth in the shortest time possible.

What you should expect from this program

1. You may get stretch marks on your biceps, depending on how elastic your skin is. This is individual for everyone so that isn't guaranteed. Keep in mind that any stretch marks you get will fade over time. Your muscles may grow faster than your skin can adjust. Do you want to be pretty or do you want to be muscular and strong?

2. You will be very sore, and you may have some tendon pain for the first few workouts as your body adjusts to the extreme workloads and volume.

3. Incredible vein popping pumps.

4. Initially you may notice that some of the weight you can use on your other lifts goes down, but this is just temporary. Your body will adjust.

5. You may think that this program is not working but it is. Stick with it and get stronger than your friends!

6. **You may want to do more arm work but do not! You will get enough arm stimulation in this program and from your other lifts, pull-ups, lat pull downs, bench-press, etc.... Your arms will grow, and they will need the rest to recuperate for the next session.**

7. Confidence, strength, power, and arms that people envy, fear, and respect!

Diet and Nutrition

This book is not about diet and nutrition as there are many more and better books on that subject. However, I did want to supply some simple guidelines here that will help you out while you are on this program.

I broke this chapter up into 3 sections so you can choose the section's that will work best for you. Every person will need to read and apply the general section and one of the other sections. Only you will know which one of the other's that you need to read. Hey if you do not know, take a look in the mirror. If you are a little soft, then follow the guidelines for those people that are jolly, and if you are a hard gainer (skinny as a rail as my mother used to say), then follow the guidelines in that section. If you are too skinny or really thin, I want you to feed yourself enough healthy calories to repair and grow from the intense workout sessions ahead.

I want you to grow, not get fat so pay attention.

General dietary guidelines

1. Eliminate salt from your diet. Salt causes water retention, which can cause you to bloat.

This includes eating foods that come prepackaged and include a lot of sodium. Rule of thumb here is that if something includes over 10% of your RDA for salt, don't eat it! Watch the salt in any kind of packaged foods or soup and avoid those foods if at all possible. Remember, salt is in almost everything we eat or drink. Even raw vegetables have some salt in them.

2. Drink 10 – 8-ounce glasses of pure water every day in addition to any other liquids that you drink.

You need to stay hydrated and remember that your body is largely made up of water.

3. You want to try to consume 50 grams of protein over and beyond your bodyweight.

This will provide your arms the nutrients (amino acids) needed to rebuild the muscle. For example, if you weigh 170 lbs., then you should aim to get 220 grams of protein per day in your diet. If you weigh 130 lbs., then 180 grams of protein is needed. More is ok, but not really needed. You can get your protein from fish, eggs, beef, chicken, pork, tofu, soy protein, protein powders, protein bars, rattlesnake, or even squirrel. I don't care where you get it, just that you consume this amount every day. Ideally you will want to split up your protein throughout the day into equal or approximately equal portions. If I needed 200 grams of protein throughout the day, I could split that into 5 servings of 40 grams each. Take your protein needs in grams and split that up over 5 servings spaced out every 3 hours. Grams/5 = amount at each consumption.

4. Eat at least one meal a day that includes raw spinach, raw broccoli, raw romaine lettuce, or raw field greens.

Yes, I want you to eat something green. I usually try to eat a large spinach salad every day. Spinach has been shown to help your body produce testosterone. Testosterone helps you build muscle. Greens also provide nutrients that our bodies need and fiber to help us move all of that protein we will be eating through our body. If spinach bothers you just eat a large portion of a green cruciferous vegetable. Raw is best, but you can also steam them.

5. Eat only good carbs (low glycemic index carbs)

You want to eat good carbs only like rice, potatoes, or beans. Avoid bread and pasta, or any processed carbohydrates. If in doubt as to the carbohydrates, then look at the nutrition label.

6. Get at least 8 hours of sleep each night.

Ok, so this one doesn't have anything to do with your diet, but I wanted to get it in the plan anyway. Remember you grow when you are resting and not when you are sleeping so get those ZZZ's in!

For those that need to trim back on their stomach fat (or Big guys need love too!)

Add these guidelines in addition to the General guidelines described above.

1. Cut any caloric beverages from your diet.

That's right, diet soda only. I'll make a deal with you though and that is for every 30 minutes of intense cardio that you do each day, you can have 1 – 12-ounce soda (any kind you want). If you don't want to do 30 minutes of intense cardio, then you shouldn't drink the soda. Intense cardio is cardio where you cannot carry on a conversation because you are panting like a dog. The only exception to this rule is when you make your protein shake or my Massive Biceps and Triceps nutrient shake.

2. Next eliminate any carbohydrates consumed after 4 pm.

When you consume carbohydrates, your body releases insulin in response to that. Insulin basically helps your body process the sugar and convert it into energy that is then stored in the cell. That is great, but that grossly oversimplified and brief process that I just described can make you fat.

When protein is consumed on the other hand and you don't eat carbs, your body releases a hormone called glucagon. Glucagon causes the cells to release their stored energy. If this is done often enough your body starts using that energy (melting fat) and you get more cut. Don't worry; you can start on carbs again in the morning. Just don't eat any after 4 pm. If it is after 4 pm, skip the rice, and instead eat twice the amount of green cruciferous vegetables.

Here are some dining examples. Baked and skinless chicken breast (or two) with raw or steamed broccoli (butter buds if you must!). Or baked salmon with steamed asparagus. Or spinach salad with ranch dressing (fat free ranch preferred) and a protein shake.

3. Eliminate fats from your diet other than what is consumed and naturally found in animal protein.

For your last two meals of the day eat something like baked skinless chicken breast and steamed broccoli. I know it is boring, but you need to understand that you will have to sacrifice to get cut. Your body needs fat, but you already have enough for your body to use. Additionally, you will get enough fat in your diet with the animal proteins you are consuming.

4. Consume 1 protein drink daily in place of 1 meal.

Any protein powder will suffice. Just drink 1 daily. If you don't want to spend money on protein powder, then drink my Massive Biceps and Triceps Nutrient shake.

5. Add some cardio into your program.

If you are already doing cardio, then fantastic! Otherwise, add at least a 15-minute walk each day to your weightlifting program.

For the bean poles or those people that can't seem to gain weight (The hated minority.)

1. Get a good balance of protein, carbohydrates, and fat at each meal.

Your plate should be ¼ protein, ¼ carbohydrates, and ½ green vegetables. You should skip any junk food that is void of nutrients. I want you to eat good wholesome food and I want you to eat often.

2. Don't skip any meals.

I want you to eat 5 meals each day spaced no more than 3 hours apart. Don't skip any meals. You may find it difficult initially to eat like this, but don't skip any meals. If you absolutely have to skip solid food because you are full, then drink an additional Massive Biceps and Triceps nutrient shake in place of 1 meal.

3. Consume at least 1 protein drink daily in addition to your meals.

Any protein powder will suffice. Just drink at least 1 daily in addition to your meals. Drink 2 daily if you can stomach all of that food. If you really want to grow, set your alarm for 2 AM or 3 AM to wake up and consume a shake before returning to bed. If you don't want to spend money on protein powder, then drink my Massive Biceps and Triceps Nutrient shake.

Massive Biceps and Triceps Nutrient Shake recipe:

There is nothing unique about this recipe other than it provides you with a near perfect ratio of carbs, fat, and protein to give you a complete meal. Additionally, it gives you a great mixture of nutrients to help you recover from your workouts.

It tastes fantastic! The ingredients are readily available anywhere, it is easy to make, and the ingredients are inexpensive. What more could you ask for?

You can substitute this drink for a protein shake, and you can consume this drink multiple times during the day if needed. I still want you to eat solid food though!

1 – plastic container of yogurt – blueberry, strawberry, or vanilla taste best to me (I recommend Greek yogurt as it contains less sugar and more protein than other types of yogurt). A single serving container of yogurt is typically 6 to 8 ounces.
1 – medium banana – peeled of course!
8 – ounces of milk. My husky (chubby) friends need to use fat free skim milk and the skinny guys can use 2% milk. There is absolutely no reason for anyone to drink whole milk in my opinion, but the hard gainer folks can drink that in their shakes if desired.

Yes, you can substitute another liquid if you don't like milk, but that liquid must contain at least 6 ounces of protein per 8 ounce serving. Examples are soy milk, almond milk, and rice milk. I personally don't get along with regular milk, so I have started drinking lactose free fat free milk and that seems to solve any digestion issues I had with regular milk.

Add all of the ingredients above to a blender with some ice; blend it up until it is smooth and drink it down.

Expanded Bonus Content - Intermittent Fasting or IF:

I decided to include this chapter on Intermittent Fasting or I.F. because it has been so successfully used by people in my life, including myself. It really is revolutionary the changes that it can make in your life.

**Note 1: If you are underweight, or very thin, you do not need to use I.F., and I do not recommend it for those that are underweight.

**Note 2: I am not a doctor, and this is not to be taken as medical advice. Follow the guidelines in this chapter at your own risk, and only after consulting with your doctor.

I.F. has a myriad of benefits and some of those are listed below.

1. I.F. has been shown to reduce your insulin levels and to increase your levels of human growth hormone (HGH).
   a. Decreasing your insulin levels can help reduce your progress towards hyperinsulinemia. Hyperinsulinemia is a medical condition where your body has an excess amount of insulin in relation to the amount of glucose in the body. This condition can and does lead to insulin resistance. Insulin resistance is often a precursor to pre-diabetes, or diabetes.

b. Increasing your growth hormone has many benefits to a thin, youthful, and muscular body. HGH is a hormone produced by your pituitary gland. Bodybuilders and strength athletes have used exogeneous sources of HGH for many years to get big and strong. Using exogeneous (external) sources of HGH can be dangerous and can cause severe side effects. However, managing/manipulating your body through your diet and exercise program to produce extra HGH is typically very safe. HGH can help maintain your lean muscle mass, help build, and even repair muscle after intense exercise sessions. HGH has been shown to increase your lean muscle mass, help you burn fat, and even boost your overall resting metabolic rate.

2. I.F. has been shown to "enhance brain functioning and cognitive development" (Citation inset below). Multiple published studies have shown that I.F. can enhance brain structures and cognitive functioning. Citation inset below. Imagine having that "brain fog" lifted by fasting! I myself have experienced greatly improved clarity while in a fasted state. It really is quite amazing!

Li, Liaoliao et al. "Chronic intermittent fasting improves cognitive functions and brain structures in mice." PloS one vol. 8,6 e66069. 3 Jun. 2013, doi:10.1371/journal.pone.0066069

3. I.F. has been shown to increase autophagy. Autophagy means "self-eating" and is a process that your body uses to destroy and replace unhealthy or ill functioning components of your body at the cellular level. This is your body's way of cleaning house, so to speak. So non-functioning or dysfunctional components of the cell are broken down and replaced. This is actually a survival mechanism. Autophagy can help destroy estrogen in your body to allow more testosterone (for increased muscle) and make you

healthier in the process. The easiest way to tap into and multiply this natural process is through fasting. Scientists believe that this process can start as early as 12 hours into the fasting process, and usually peaks at around the 72-hour mark. Not only can this process help your body and muscle building, but it can also help your brain perform at peak capacity. Think about this, once your body believes it is in starvation mode it has one function, to find food. Your body begins this process to keep you going in your quest to do just that. There have been multiple reports of people reversing disease by following fasting protocols, and there are even clinics in Russia that have extremely strict and long fasting programs.

Now, I know what you are thinking… All that sounds great, but how do I do it? The process is quite simple. You will just have an eating window and a non-eating window.

During the non-eating window, you will not consume any calories. Non-caloric beverages are fine (water, diet soda, Crystal light, unsweetened tea, black coffee, etc.…), just no solid food or anything with calories.

During the eating window you will consume healthy and nutritional food as you normally would.

That is, it. Simple, isn't it?

I have personally fasted for 10 days, while only consuming, less than 500 calories a day. This is rather extreme though, and I wouldn't recommend it unless you can severely limit all physical activities during this time. With extreme and long-term fasting, always get guidance from a medical doctor that is familiar with your health conditions.

Most people struggle a little bit with I.F. the first couple of days, but your body very quickly adapts to this new circumstance. Next, we will dive into some of the very simple Fasting protocols that most people use.

Easiest method for most people – 16X8 - I.F.

The easiest method for most people is to start their fast after dinner and carry it forward into the morning. Some people skip breakfast anyway, and most people don't eat during the night so for most this is the easiest method.

This method is known as the 16X8 method. Basically, it allows you to have a 16-hour non-eating window and an 8-hour eating window in a given day. This is the method I use most often because I find it the least disruptive to my working and family schedule. You can use this method every day.

Here is how it typically works. On this program you would finish dinner by 7:00 pm (adjust as needed for eating window), begin fasting, sleep, skip breakfast, and then eat your first meal (for me this is lunch) usually at 11:00 am. Then you could eat as normally until 7:00 pm. Then repeat the process over again.

If you eat at different times, for example, if you work the night shift, just adjust the associated eating window so that all food (all calories) are consumed in an 8-hour window. You will be a little hungry for the first few days until your body adjusts to the new schedule.

What seems to help me best, when I fall off the wagon, and need to get back into it, is to do at least 1 week of very low carb dieting prior to starting. This reduces my sugar cravings and helps me control my appetite. This, in turn, makes starting the fasting very easy.
Please note that as your fasting becomes more "extreme" your results will accelerate.

Keep in mind, that as your schedule changes, your eating window can also change, as long as you maintain the fasted time. So, if you have to eat earlier or later one day, just factor that into calculating your next eating window.

A little bit more challenging method for most people is to limit their eating window to a 4-hour timeframe. This method is known as the 20X4 method. Using this method, you will have a non-eating, or fasting window of 20 hours each day, followed by a 4-hour eating window. This allows you to eat 1 large meal each day with possibly a couple of protein shakes, or 2 smaller meals with only 1 protein shake.

Sometimes people start with the 16X8 method and then transition to the 20X4 I.F. if they want to speed up their progress and as their body adjusts to intermittent fasting.

This method will accelerate your results significantly. Especially since you will typically be performing all exercise during the fasting window which will force your body to burn additional fat.

Keep in mind, that as your schedule changes, your eating window can also change, as long as you maintain the fasted time. So, if you have to eat earlier or later one day, just factor that into calculating your next eating window.

Let me provide you with some sample schedules below.

Sample option 1 – with 1 small to medium sized meal and 2 supplemental snacks/shakes
- Get off of work at 5:00 pm.
- Have a protein, meal replacement, or MB&T Nutrient shake on the way to the gym.
- Finish your workout and eat dinner 6:30 pm – 7:30 pm.

- Consume a protein, meal replacement, of MB&T Nutrient shake by 9:00 pm
- Eating window 5:00 pm – 9:00 pm

Sample option 2 – with 1 medium to large meal and 1 supplemental snacks/shakes
- Get off of work at 5:00 pm.
- Have a protein, meal replacement, or MB&T Nutrient shake on the way to the gym.
- Finish your workout by – 7:30 pm.
- Consume a medium to large meal and finish eating by 9:00 pm.

Sample option 3 – with 2 small meals and 1 supplemental snacks/shakes
- Get off of work at 5:00 pm.
- Consume a small and nutritionally balanced meal on the way to the gym.
- Finish your workout - 6:30 pm
- Have a protein, meal replacement, or MB&T Nutrient shake, post workout.
- Consume another small meal and finish eating by 9:00 pm.

Also keep in mind you can switch between a 16X8 and a 20X4 method. I will sometimes do this depending on my schedule. For example, if I know I am going to have a very intense workout day, I may do the 16X8 on the day of my workout to ensure that my body has the nutrients it needs. Then on my rest day I will revert back to the 20X4 fasting method.

Also, let's say that I know I will be a glutton on a given date (Thanksgiving, Christmas, a certain Las Vegas buffet that I can't resist, or a certain Brazilian steakhouse…) I will switch to the 20X4 method, eat the gigantic meal, and not be impacted by it as severely because that meal will be the only thing, I eat that day.

You can really customize any of these options for what makes sense to you and feels right for your body.

24 hour - 36 hour - I.F.

This is the most extreme and most challenging fasting method that I will recommend in this book. This method maximizes autophagy, and produces the fastest weight loss, while minimizing any associated health risks. Other methods certainly exist, but I will not recommend them because I believe they can be very detrimental to gaining muscle mass and strength.

Using these methods, you avoid consuming any calories at all for 24 hours up to 36 hours.

Some scientific research has shown that you can consume up to 500 calories during these "fasting" windows and still maintain your fasted state. However, I have found that once I break the fast, I am not able to restrict my caloric intake to 500 or below calories and that this destroys any progress I have made. Your mileage may vary.

Here is the easiest way I have found to do this. I eat a very large breakfast on Saturday morning finishing by 9:00 am. This will keep me feeling full for several hours. I then consume no additional calories until breakfast after 9:00 am on Sunday (24-hours). If I can extend that time, all the better.

This is easy for me, because I am not working on Saturday evening typically, so if I am hungry or hangry, I can just relax, drink some iced tea, and enjoy family time. Sunday mornings are the days that my family typically sleeps in so hitting the eating window after 9:00 am, is no big deal. We also go to church on Sunday, so oftentimes, my fasting window gets extended to 1:00 pm (28-hours) or 2:00 pm (29-hours) on Sunday when the family and I go have lunch after church. Sometimes with driving to the location, ordering, etc.… it may be 4:00 pm (31-hours), before a morsel of food touches my lips.

If I can extend the fasted time, then even better. Sometimes I do extend the time if I am not hungry. Sometimes I follow this schedule on Sunday itself, and then start eating on Monday.

This sounds harder and harsher than it is. The first time you do it, it can be challenging (more mental than physical), but it will get easier, and actually it is kind of exciting to know that you can miss 1, 2, or several meals and be fine. Before too long, you will even be able to have pleasant chats with people that are eating, even though you are fasting.

Modern society has made us too impatient and weak regarding food. We all want instant gratification which is why you can find so many food vendors and fast food restaurants on every corner.

I hope this section on Intermittent Fasting helps you reach your fitness and life goals! Good luck to you!

Equipment needed

To put it simply, not much; that is what makes this program so beautiful. You will however need a few items, and I have listed those below. For the barbell curls you can use either a straight bar or an ez-curl bar, but I prefer straight bars.

Item	Quantity of Item
Barbell or Ez-Curl bar – the one that can accept weight plates, not the ones that have a fixed weight.	1
Dumbbells – preferably the ones that can accept weight plates. The dumbbell bars with collars should each weigh about 5 pounds.	2
Weight plates	Lots of plates, from 2.5 lbs. to 45 lbs.
Small weight plates or weighted gloves with a combined weight no more than 3 lbs.	2 – 1.25 or 1.5 lb. plates or 2 – 1.5 lb. weighted gloves (more on this later)
Weightlifting belt – (optional, but never a bad idea)	1
Flat bench	1
A stopwatch, the timer on your phone, or some other type of time keeping device.	1 used to record rest periods and wrist twisting times.

Determination and an indomitable spirit	1

The Exercises

These are the only acceptable exercises for this program. No substitutions are allowed.

Biceps Exercises

Wrist twists with empty dumbbells – arms straight

This exercise serves to warm up your wrists and forearms for the workout ahead. This exercise also pre-fatigues your forearm muscles and primes them for the rest of the exercises. Ideally you will use heavy, and empty dumbbell bars with the collars on (if they are the screw on collars).

You can also use a heavy pipe for this exercise as well, just make sure it is 10 to 15 inches long and has a weight of between 3 and 5 lbs.

To perform the exercise, grasp the dumbbell bars in the center, one in each hand. Extend your arms out to your sides. Your hands should be about 18 inches from your body with your arms straight. Grip the bars as tightly as you can (like you are trying to break them) and twist them rapidly back and forth as quickly as possible. You should try to get 1 twist back and forth each second. Continue this back and forth twisting for 1 minute straight with no breaks or stoppages.

Wrist twists with empty dumbbells – arms bent at 90 degrees

This exercise is very similar to the Wrist twists with empty dumbbells – arms straight exercise with the exception that your arms are bent at the elbow into a 90-degree angle.

To perform the exercise, grasp dumbbell bars in the center, one in each hand. Extend your arms out to your sides. Now bend your elbow so that your forearm is at a 90-degree angle to your biceps muscle. Your forearm should be parallel to the floor. Grip the bars as tightly as you can (like you are trying to break them) and twist them rapidly back and forth as quickly as possible. You should try to get 1 twist back and forth each second. Continue this back and forth twisting for 1 minute straight with no breaks or stoppages.

21's

21's are not used very much anymore, but they are an awesome exercise for placing maximum stress on your biceps muscle and creating growth.

The motion used in 21's is the same as the motion for barbell curls. They are called 21's because you do 7 reps up to the halfway point of your curling motion from the bottom, then you do 7 reps from the top to the halfway point of your curling motion followed immediately by 7 full barbell curls throughout the full range of motion. 3 times 7 is 21, hence the name.

To perform this exercise, grasp a barbell (that has the appropriate amount of weight plates added to it) with a shoulder width or slightly less than shoulder width grip. Your feet should be shoulder width apart and you should be standing upright with the bar resting near your pelvis. Perform 7 controlled repetitions from the bottom up to the halfway point. Your forearms should be approximately parallel to the floor. Pause for a half second count at the stopping point. Then lower back to the bottom of the movement for the next rep. Do this for 7 repetitions.

Then curl the barbell up to the top of your range of motion (perform a barbell curl from the bottom, all the way to the top), and lower it back to the halfway point pausing for a half second count at the stopping point, before curling back up to the top. Do this for 7 repetitions.

Finally, complete the exercise by curling the weight from the bottom, to the top of your range of motion in a controlled manner. Pay attention to your form and maintain good form throughout the entire movement. Do 7 full curls, all the way up and then back down.

Dumbbell Hammer Curls

This is a great exercise for your forearms and hits your biceps brachii muscle. It also works your brachialis muscle, which will lift your biceps brachii giving your flexed muscle more height.

To perform this exercise, load 2 dumbbells (with the appropriate amount of weight plates added to each) with the same amount of weight. For example, each dumbbell could be loaded with 30, 40, or 50 lbs. Pick the appropriate weight for you and make certain that you use the same amount of weight on each dumbbell. Your feet should be shoulder width apart and you should be standing upright with each dumbbell resting on your side near your hip.

Holding each dumbbell as you would a hammer, curl each hand up to the top of your range of motion. Hold for a half second count before lowering each dumbbell back to the starting position.

Alternating Dumbbell Curls

The alternating dumbbell curl is a good way to correct any strength and size imbalances in the biceps as it works each muscle individually. In this exercise you will alternate the curling movement with each arm.

To perform this exercise, load 2 dumbbells (with the appropriate amount of weight plates added to each) with the same amount of weight. For example, each dumbbell could be loaded with 30, 40, or 50 lbs. Pick the appropriate weight for you and make certain that you use the same amount of weight on each dumbbell. Your feet should be shoulder width apart and you should be standing upright with each dumbbell resting near your side near your hip. Palms should be up, and you should hold the dumbbells as if you were doing a barbell curl.

Your palms should be facing up, with the dumbbells not touching your body. Before starting the set, take up the slack by lifting up the weight slightly so the tension is on your bicep muscles. Starting with your weakest arm (usually the left), curl the dumbbell up as far as possible. Squeeze the bicep at the top of the exercise, and then slowly lower the weight down without it touching your body or taking the tension off your bicep. Repeat that motion with the other arm. That is one repetition (rep). Now repeat for the desired amount of reps, alternating the movement arm to arm.

Reverse Barbell Curls

This movement works the brachioradialis muscle as well as the biceps muscle and is important to develop overall arm strength.

To perform this exercise, stand with your knees slightly bent, while holding a barbell with your hands palm down. Your hands should be about shoulder width apart. Without heaving your shoulders, whipping your arms, or snapping the muscles taught, lift the weight until it touches your upper chest. Your elbows should come slightly forward as you lift, but they should not move out sideways. Then lower the bar back down so that it rests at your pelvis level. Repeat for the desired number of reps.

Concentration Curls

The dumbbell concentration curl will specifically target your biceps muscle to achieve a maximum contraction.

To perform this exercise, sit on a chair or your flat bench with feet placed comfortably apart somewhat wider than the shoulder and with the feet and lower legs angled slightly outward. Hold a dumbbell in one hand with that arm hanging down between your legs and next to the thigh of the same side leg. Bend over at the waist yet with the back as straight as possible and not curved over. Get ready to curl the dumbbell up and then down between your legs. You need some space for this.
Brace the rear of the upper arm against the inside of the thigh above the knee while holding the dumbbell in the lowered position. Curl the dumbbell upward then down again, ensuring the rear of the upper arm is firmly braced against the thigh. That is one rep. Repeat for the desired number of reps. Then switch arms and perform the same number of reps for the other arm.

Barbell Curls

This exercise is the basic movement to build your biceps muscles. Everyone knows how to do this one.

To perform this exercise, stand with your knees slightly bent, while holding a barbell with your hands palms up. Your hands should be about shoulder width apart. Without heaving your shoulders, whipping your arms, or snapping the muscles taught, lift the weight until it touches your upper chest or comes close to touching your upper chest. Your elbows should come slightly forward as you lift, but they should not move out sideways. Keep your elbows locked to your sides. Then lower the bar back down so that it rests at your pelvis level. Repeat for the desired number of reps.

Triceps Exercises

Close Grip Push-ups

This exercise is used in the routines to pre-fatigue the triceps muscles. Once they are fatigued, the heavy work sets are started to maximize muscle activation. This exercise also strengthens the connective tissue in your arm and especially your elbow joint.

To perform this exercise, assume a push-up position on the floor. Your hands should be directly under and slightly higher than chest level. Keep your hands a maximum of 6 inches apart. If you are strong enough, you can touch your index fingers and thumbs together so that the space between your hands creates a triangle. Lift yourself up off of the ground using your triceps muscles to push you. You should feel maximum stress in your triceps and in your elbow joint. Hold the position at the top for a half second count, and slowly lower your chest back down to the floor. That is one rep. Modifications to this exercise can be doing the push-ups off of your knees instead of the toes of your feet. Also, you can move your hands apart up to 6 inches to lower the stress felt. However, you should always try to work toward keeping your hands together and performing the push-up from the toes of your feet. Repeat for the desired number of reps.

Bench Dips

Bench dips will pack on slabs of muscle to your triceps and will also strengthen your chest and your front deltoid.

To perform these exercises, sit on a bench so that your body and the bench form a T shape. Slowly scoot your bottom off of the bench and grab the bench with your hands to hold you up. Your hands should be on the edge of the bench right next to your hips.

You should be hanging off of the bench and holding yourself up with your hands. Your feet and legs should be placed closely together and on the ground in front of you. Keep your legs straight throughout the movement. Keeping your back straight, slowly lower yourself down as so that your upper arm is parallel to the ground. Hold for a half second count at the bottom of the movement before pushing yourself back up. Squeeze your triceps muscles at the top. You should feel this movement in your triceps if you are doing it correctly. Be careful not to completely lock out your elbows at the top. You should be about half an inch from locking out your elbows. Hold for a half second count at the top and then repeat for the desired number of reps.

French Curls or Skull crushers

This movement adds size, strength and definition to your triceps muscle.

To perform this exercise, lie on a bench with your feet touching the floor, and grasp the barbell (that is loaded with the appropriate weight). Push the barbell over your head. Lock your elbows/arms into your side and be sure to perform the movement with only your elbows bending. The barbell should be over your forehead, hence the name, skull crushers. Keep your hands about 8 but no more than 10 inches apart. Keep your upper arms stationary, slowly lower the barbell down so that it touches or almost touches your forehead. Hold for a half second count and then push it back up to the top of your range, using your triceps muscles. That completes one rep. Repeat for the desired number of reps.

Triceps Kickbacks

This is a serious sculpting movement for your entire triceps muscle.

Stand to the right of your weight bench, holding a dumbbell in your right hand with your palm facing into your side. Place your left lower leg (the area directly under your knee) and your left hand on top of the bench. Bend forward at the hips until your upper body is bent over the bench at a 45-degree angle to the floor. Bend your right elbow so your upper arm is parallel to the floor, your forearm is perpendicular to it, and your palm faces in. Keep your elbow close to your waist. Pay attention that your arm stays pinned into your waist and does not move down with each movement. Bend your knees slightly. Keeping your upper arm still and pinned to your side, straighten your arm behind you until your entire arm is parallel to the floor and one end of the dumbbell points toward the floor. Squeeze the triceps muscle at the top. Hold for a half second count, and then slowly bend your arm to lower the weight. That completes one repetition. Repeat for the desired number of reps. When you complete the set, repeat the exercise with your left arm.

The Rules

I know, I hate rules too, but if you want sleeve-busting arms you are going to have to follow the rules.

Measure your arm with a Tailor's tape measure. They are cheap and you can buy one almost anywhere.

A Tailor's or cloth tape measure is flexible and is used to measure the circumference and length of body parts like your inseam.

Use the tape measure to measure the circumference of your upper arm both in the flexed (the tape should fit over the largest portion of your arm which includes the head of your bicep) and relaxed states. Record the circumference from both measurements because you will want to measure both again at the end of this program.

1. Calculate your 10-rep maximum on the barbell curl. Don't do this on a machine. I'm talking about a barbell loaded with weight plates. The weight selected should allow you to curl cleanly without slinging the weight and screaming like a 12-year-old girl that just met Justin Bieber.

You should be able to complete 10 reps without failure or compromising your form.

2. I'm not going to teach you how to do a barbell curl; there are a million sites on the Internet that can teach you how to do that. Bodybuilding.com is a good site to look up the exercises on if you are search engine challenged.

3. Take that 10-rep max weight number, whatever it is, and write it down. You will use that number in the next calculation.

4. Now multiply your 10-rep max by .7. You will be using 70% of your 10-rep max for one of the biceps routines. If the routine is too hard, you can drop that to 60%, but I want you to resist the urge to do that if at all possible. For example, if you would be using 100 pounds for 10-reps, then your weight would be 70 lbs.

5. Next take that 10-rep max number and multiply it by 1.25. You will be using 125 % of your 10-rep max for the other bicep's routine. If the routine is too hard, you can drop that to 120%, but I want you to resist the urge to do that if at all possible. For example, if you would be using 100 pounds for 10-reps, then your weight would be 125 lbs.

6. Now write down 40% of your weight that was recorded in Step 4. Round up the weight if needed. For example, if you are using 70lbs. from step 4. 70 X .4 = 28 lbs. I would be using 28 lbs. to start for my other lifts in the bicep's routine. If you don't have the weight plates to create this weight round up to the nearest value, you can match. For example, if you can't create 28lbs. with your current weight plates you round the weight up to 30 lbs. or down to 25 lbs.

7. Finally record 60% of the number from step 4, to use as your starting weight for French curls. For example, if you were using 70 lbs. from step 4, then you would use 42 lbs. on this number. If you don't have the weight plates to create this weight round up or down to the nearest value, you can match.

8. Resist the urge to alter the program or to go off of it.

9. Every time you do the biceps routines and triceps routine in this program, I want you to increase the weight by 2.5 lbs. This is where the small weight plates (1.25lbs.) or weighted gloves come in. I want you to do this on every exercise where indicated in the routines located in this book.

The Routines

The Massive Biceps and Triceps program is comprised of 2 Biceps routines and 1 Triceps routine. You will only work out your arms on this program twice each week. I don't care if you don't think that is enough. That is all you will do on this program.

Believe in the program and you will see results.

Each Biceps routine will be used 1 time each week and you will immediately follow the Biceps routine with the Triceps routine. You will alternate the Biceps routines, beginning with Biceps routine 1 on program day 1, then doing Biceps routine 2 on the next day that you work your arms, then back to Biceps routine 1 and so on until your 30 day program is over.

Do no other arm work other than what is specified in this program.

Stretch your biceps and triceps thoroughly before each workout.

Biceps Routine 1

This program employs supersets to increase hypertrophy in the target muscle group. You will not rest between sets, but instead flow directly into the next exercise.

Exercise	Goal/Sets & Reps
Wrist twists arms straight	1 minute
No rest	
Wrist twists arms bent	1 minute
21's	1 set of 21 reps, using the weight recorded in Step 4 of The Rules section. * Up in weight by 2.5 lbs. the next time you perform this exercise.
Dumbbell Hammer Curls	8 reps using the weight recorded in Step 6 of The Rules section. * Up in weight by 2.5 lbs. the next time you perform this exercise.
Alternating Dumbbell Curls	8 reps using the weight recorded in Step 6 of The Rules section. * Up in weight by 2.5 lbs. the next time you perform this exercise.

Reverse Barbell Curls	8 reps using the weight recorded in Step 6 + 10 pounds. * Up in weight by 2.5 lbs. the next time you perform this exercise.
Concentration Curls	8 reps using the weight recorded in Step 6 of The Rules section. * Up in weight by 2.5 lbs. the next time you perform this exercise.

* If you do not have the weight plates to increase the weight by 2.5 lbs. you can add your weighted gloves. For example, the first time I do this routine, I use my recorded weights from The Rules section without my weighted gloves. The second time I perform this routine; I use my weighted gloves and the weight recorded from The Rules section. The third time I perform this routine, I add 5 lbs. to the weights recorded in The Rules section, and I do not use the weighted gloves. This process continues until I complete the program.

Biceps Routine 2

This routine forces your body into muscle confusion
because you are lifting more weight than you normally do.
This results in maximizing the stress on the biceps muscle
and the adaptive response of the body. It employs rest to
ensure that you are ready for the next set.

Exercise	Goal/Sets & Reps
Wrist twists arms straight	1 minute
No rest	
Wrist twists arms bent	1 minute
Barbell Curls	10 sets of 3 repetitions each set. Use the weight recorded in Step 5 of The Rules section. * Move up in weight by 2.5 lbs. the next time you do this routine. Rest for 1 full minute between sets. Use your weight belt for this routine!

* If you do not have the weight plates to increase the
weight by 2.5 lbs. you can add your weighted gloves. For

example, the first time I do this routine, I use my recorded weights from The Rules section without my weighted gloves. The second time I perform this routine; I use my weighted gloves and the weight recorded from The Rules section. The third time I perform this routine, I add 5 lbs. to the weights recorded in The Rules section, and I do not use the weighted gloves. This process continues until I complete the program.

Triceps Routine

This routine pushes your triceps to exhaustion raising the level of training stress on the triceps muscle group. The timing and range of motion in this routine work synergistically to maximize the adaptive response of your body causing your triceps to grow. This routine also strengthens your tendons in your arm.

Exercise	Goal/Sets & Reps
Close Grip Push-ups	10 – 15 reps using your body weight
No rest	
Bench Dips	2 sets of 12 – 15 reps using your body weight. Rest for 1 full minute between sets. * You can add a small amount of weight on your lap for this exercise once you meet the set and rep count, but it is not necessary. **Move directly from this exercise to the next with only the amount of rest it takes you to grab the barbell and**

	lay down on the bench.
French Curls or Skull crushers	3 sets of 8 – 12 reps using the weight recorded in Step 7 of The Rules section. Rest for 1 full minute between sets. * Move up in weight by 2.5 lbs. as soon as you can get 3 sets of 12 reps. **Do not rest on the last set but move directly to Kickbacks**

Triceps Kickbacks	2 sets of 12 – 15 reps using 10 lb. dumbbells to start. If 10 lbs. seemed too light, the next time bump the weight up to 15 or 20 lbs. until you find the **correct weight.** *Move up in weight by 2.5 lbs. each time you do this routine from the correct weight. Do not rest between sets, as you will already be alternating arms when performing sets. One arm will rest as the other arm is working.

* If you do not have the weight plates to increase the weight by 2.5 lbs. you can add your weighted gloves.

The Schedule

How much and how often should you do this program? This program is a 4-week program designed to greatly accelerate your upper arm development. This means that you should workout using my program a total of 8 times in 30 days.

After this program, I would recommend that you go back to a standard weight-training program for at least 6 weeks to allow your body time to recover before beginning my program again if desired.

At the end of this program you should anticipate new size, strength, and development in your upper arms. Don't take my word for it though, recalculate your new 10-rep maximum and take your new arm measurements!

When you do the program will depend on your current workout schedule. I recommend that you only do the **Massive Biceps and Triceps (MB&T)** program 2 times per week.

You should allow at least 2 days of rest between each session and 3 days is even better. This routine will maximally stress your body.

I have attempted to put a schedule below that will fit with most of your weight training programs. If it doesn't, you can customize it but don't do my program more than twice each week. Doing that won't lead to better or quicker results.

Alternate Biceps Routines on every workout day (e.g., Biceps Routine 1, then Biceps Routine 2, then back to Biceps Routine 1). Immediately followed by the Triceps routine.

Again, do not do any other arm workout or arm exercises other than my program for the full 30 days!

Whole body 3 day per week split.

Monday	Wednesday	Friday
Whole Body workout	Whole Body workout	Whole Body workout
MB&T -Biceps Routine 1 -Triceps Routine	**No arm work**	**MB&T** - Biceps Routine 2 - Triceps Routine

Four day per week split (each body part two times each week).

Day of the Week	Routine
Monday	Lower body work
Tuesday	Upper body work ------ plus----- **MB&T** Biceps Routine 1 Triceps Routine
Wednesday	Rest day
Thursday	Lower body work
Friday	Upper body work ------ plus----- **MB&T** Biceps Routine 2 Triceps Routine
Saturday	Rest day

Six day per week split.

Day of the Week	Routine
Monday	Lower body work
Tuesday	Upper body work ------ plus----- **MB&T** Biceps Routine 1 Triceps Routine
Wednesday	Lower body work
Thursday	Upper body work ------ plus----- ****No additional or specific arm work. For example, bent-over rows or lat pulldowns are okay, but no exercises that specifically target your biceps or triceps.**
Friday	Lower body work
Saturday	Upper body work ------ plus----- **MB&T** Biceps Routine 2 Triceps Routine
Sunday	Rest day

Thank you

I want to personally thank each one of you for trusting this program and me.

You are in charge of your destiny and we should all strive to be the best people that we can be on a mental, physical, and spiritual level. You have taken a great step toward making your arms as muscular as they can be.

Happy lifting and enjoy your new arm size!

If you would ever like to contact me, please do so at mcnealbooks@gmail.com.

I hope that you find the information here helpful, useful, and that you meet all your goals in life.

Very Truly yours,
Justin McNeal

Closing

Dear Reader,

Every time I write a book, I get email from readers and fans thanking me for the book. Some have important feedback on how I can improve my writing, some have suggestions on future topics that I should write about, and still others just give me critical feedback about what they thought about the book. Loved it or hated it, it is important for me to know what you think.

As an author, I love feedback. Candidly, you are the primary reason that I write. So, tell me what you liked, what you loved, even what you hated. I'd love to hear from you. You can always contact me at my Blog (http://justinmcneal.blogspot.com/) or at mcnealbooks@gmail.com.

I would love to hear from you!

Finally, I need to ask you for a favor. If you are so inclined, I would love to have a review of any of my books on Amazon.com. Loved it, hated it – I would just enjoy your feedback.

As you may have noticed, reviews can be tough to come by these days. You, the reader, have the power now to make or break a book. If you would like to, please review my books (any that you have read) on Amazon.com, I would really love to hear from you.

Thank you so much for reading my book(s), for supporting me, and for spending time with me.

In sincerest gratitude,
Justin McNeal